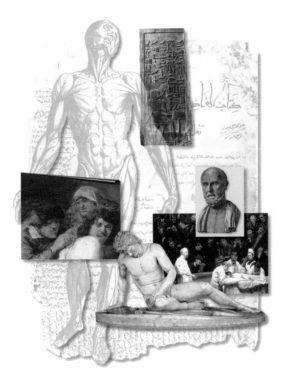

First Edition

Copyright © 1998 Ortho-McNeil Pharmaceutical, Inc. and Janssen-Cilag

Library of Congress Cataloging-in-Publication Data
A Brief History of Wound Healing/OCC Inc. editor.—1st ed.
ISBN 0-9660389-0-8
1. History—wound healing, wound care, chronic wound care.
2. Wound Healing—history, chronicle, record, account.
3. Dressings—bandages, topical wound care drugs.

OCC thanks Henry Brown, MD for his insightful comments and editorial assistance.

Published by Oxford Clinical Communications Inc., 301 Oxford Valley Road, Building 1301, Yardley, Pennsylvania, USA

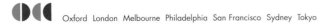

Oxford London Melbourne Philadelphia San Francisco Sydney Tokyo

ORTHO·MCNEIL   JANSSEN-CILAG

Table of Contents

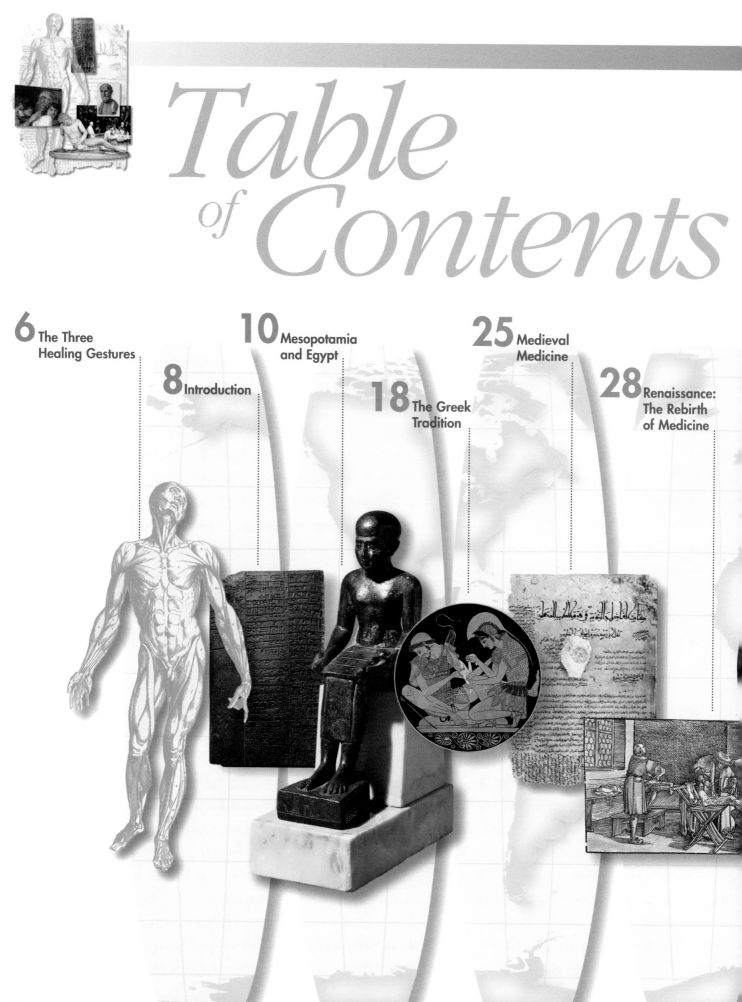

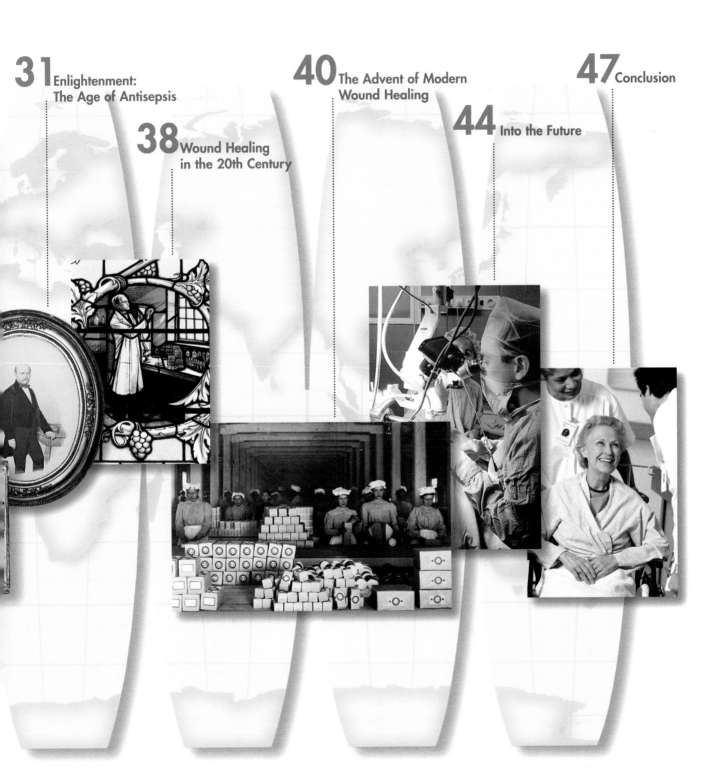

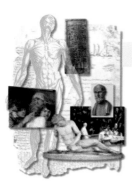

Foreword

You are about to read a concise history of wound healing. It is intended to provide you with a biopsy of the past and a glimpse into the future. Hopefully, it will inspire you to read even more about the past, as this will enhance your abilities for the future. One cannot be a leader and innovator in wound healing without an awareness of its history.

Long before any scientific tools were available, our medical forefathers made careful observations of wounds. Amazingly, either through rational thought or empiricism, they were able to develop many sound therapies for both acute and chronic wounds. This text provides some of the scientific explanations for the rationale behind these ancient therapies. In many ways, science is just beginning to catch up with and explain treatments known for centuries on an empirical basis.

What stands out is the incredible paucity of information during the Dark Ages and even during the enlightened 18th and 19th centuries. For example, for many decades the establishment refused to recognize the role of bacteria in wound sepsis and death. Those who spoke out in favor of these new ideas were often chastised and ostracized by their colleagues.

Clearly, the great clinical observers, such as Paré, Semmelweis, and Lister, to name a few, have always been the key to meaningful discoveries. At first, Fleming cursed the mold that grew on his culture dish because it impeded the growth of the bacteria he wished to study. It took 12 years, and the work of Howard Florey, Norman Heatley, and Ernst Chain, before it was recognized that the mold he cursed could be used to kill bacteria that caused wound infections in humans. And the age of antibiotics began. This example, only one of many, illustrates how we must carefully scrutinize each experiment conducted and wound observed if we are to see progress in wound healing. Some of the greatest lessons from the text that follows are to avoid being locked into tradition or hampered by current dogma.

It has only been in the past two decades that the field of wound care has received the attention it deserves from industry and caregivers. When I decided to spend time at the National Institutes of Health (NIH) in 1970 to learn more about healing, many of my surgical colleagues thought I was on a fool's mission. Gross, Peacock, Dumphy— and young Tom Hunt—were among the few investigators with laboratories or clinical programs that focused on wound healing. Today, there is a surfeit of societies, journals, meetings, and biotechnology companies devoted to studying the process of wound healing. Wounds are "in" because they represent unsolved clinical problems that often lead to long-term disability and death. Healthcare payors look for solutions to these problems to provide better, more efficient, and less expensive care.

It is exciting to witness the evolution of recent research into the use of newly designed dressings, growth factors, and various pharmacologic agents for the management of acute and chronic wounds. The proper use of growth factors is now within our grasp thanks to those in industry and academia with the foresight to direct studies designed with great care. Moreover, investigators who are looking into the contents of human wound fluids and tissue should find answers that will enhance our understanding and rationale for the more effective use of growth factors and other drugs. For example, understanding the microenvironment of the chronic wound may well lead to the use of protease inhibitors in chronic wounds. Perhaps more exciting than the work in healing chronic wounds is the potential to prevent them from ever occurring, prevent deep tissue fibrosis such as cirrhosis of the liver, and even induce regeneration of pristine tissue rather than repair of damaged tissue.

The future of wound healing appears very exciting, and this text provides an excellent guide to where we have been. Equally important, it may provide clues to get us where we would like to go, for as Santayana stated: "those who cannot remember the past are condemned to repeat it."

— *I. Kelman Cohen, MD*

The era of modern wound healing began in the 19th century with the discovery of bacteria and their role in the pathogenesis of infection. This development, however, was not an isolated event but the culmination of thousands of years of scientific and medical research.

The *Three*
Heal

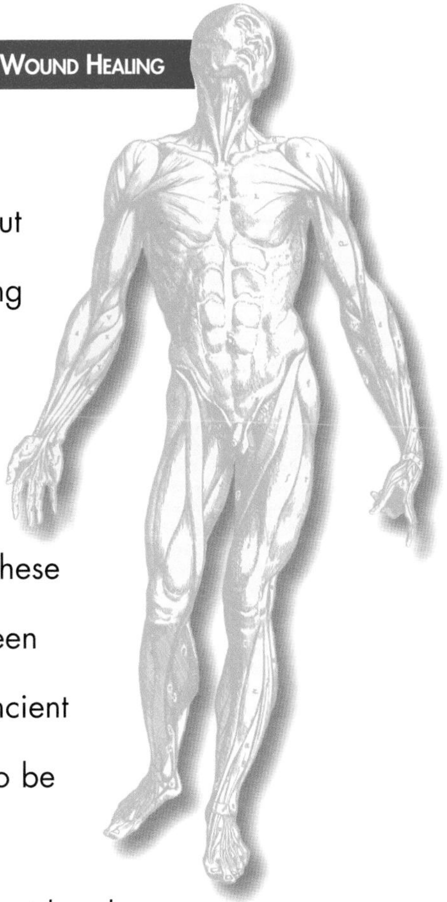

The events described in this book span several millennia and stretch from the oldest known writings to wound care as it is practiced today. The intention is not to present a comprehensive history of wound healing as such, but to provide the reader with a brief survey of some of the more relevant episodes in the history of science and medicine as they relate to wound healing.

A common theme throughout this book is the three healing gestures—what modern clinicians would call "interventions." Judging from the historical record, these gestures appear to have been practiced by most of the ancient civilizations and continue to be practiced today. The three healing gestures can be considered the thread with which the history of wound healing is woven.

" …and went to him, and bound his wounds, pouring in oil and wine "

-Luke, 10:34

" …the surface of the sick part with butter you shall anoint… "

-ancient Assyrian Medical Text

" With bandage firm, Ulysses' knee they bound "

-Homer, The Odyssey

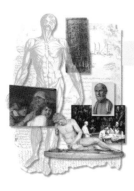

INTRODUCTION

The history of wound healing is, in a sense, the history of mankind. Unlike many less complex organisms, humans lack the ability to regenerate lost or damaged limbs. In the evolutionary process, we traded the slow biological sophistication of regeneration for relatively simple and more rapid healing. For man in the ancient world, wound care was an indispensable part of life as it is today.

Alone among animals, man has developed the ability to pass knowledge down to future generations via written symbols. So it is not surprising that some of the oldest writings recovered from archeological findings describe the care and treatment of wounds. Indeed, physician (or healer) was an occupation recognized by each of the four ancient river-valley civilizations.

One of the oldest medical manuscripts known to man is a clay tablet that dates back to circa 2200 B.C. This tablet describes, perhaps for the first time, the "three healing gestures," which consist of:

One of the oldest known medical texts is a clay tablet (circa 2200 B.C.) consisting of a collection of prescriptions.

1 washing the wound

2 making plasters

3 bandaging the wound

What the ancients and early moderns referred to as plasters are the present day equivalent of wound dressings. These are mixtures of substances applied to wounds to provide protection and to absorb exudate.

These three gestures are what we would refer to today as interventions. They appear in ancient records recovered from civilizations widely separated both geographically and temporally, and these gestures continue to be practiced today. In fact, much of the history of wound healing can be considered a variation on these three themes: (1) cleansing the wound to remove debris and control bacteria, (2) applying dressings to protect the wound from infection, and (3) bandaging the wound to protect it from re-injury and at times to prevent excessive or recurrent bleeding. Most major advances in wound healing, until the present, fall within the realm of one or more of the three healing gestures.

Throughout the ages, an amazing variety of different methods and substances have been used to treat wounds. Each method or substance was considered an improvement in one of the three healing gestures, at least by those who discovered them. Some of these wound healing substances were used as they were found in nature. Many methods involved preparation of substances that required extensive processing following recipes that were quite intricate. Recipes sometimes consisted of dozens of different ingredients, mixed in a precisely defined manner, and often requiring the assistance of a priest or magician. In contrast, some methods consisted of simply smearing mud on the wound.

Section of the Ebers papyrus (circa 1550 B.C.), discovered by Georg Ebers at Thebes in 1872. This remarkable manuscript contains protocols for the treatment of many medical conditions.

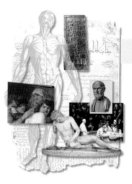

MESOPOTAMIA AND EGYPT

One of the earliest known wound care products was beer; the Sumerians brewed at least 19 different types. An ancient Mesopotamian prescription for healing a person "sick with a blow on the cheek" reads as follows:

" *...pound together fur-turpentine, pine-turpentine, tamarisk, daisy, flour of Inninnu. Strain; mix in milk and beer in a small copper pan; spread on skin, bind on him, and he shall recover.* "

Mummified head of the Pharaoh Ramses V, 1160 B.C.

Plasters were made from many different substances, including mud or clay, plants, and herbs. In addition, one of the most common ingredients used in plasters was oil. The type of oil used varied from region to region. Oil was also used as part of many religious ceremonies and was the main source of light in the ancient world. For these reasons, it had immense ritualistic value and was probably applied to wounds as part of a wound healing ritual. However, as Guido Majno points out in his book *The Healing Hand, Man and Wound in the Ancient World*, oil may have provided some protection from infection (bacteria grow poorly in oil) and prevented the bandage from sticking to the wound (nonadherent dressings).

In ancient Egypt, the art of wound healing flourished. The Greeks and later the Romans were heavily influenced by Egyptian medicine.

Egyptian civilization and the various Mesopotamian civilizations overlapped considerably in time. Even though by today's standards they were not widely separated geographically, there was little interaction between the cultures initially because they were separated by the Arabian desert. Later, when Mesopotamian influence reached the Mediterranean Sea, the two cultures intermingled.

Our knowledge of Egyptian medicine is alive today through a series of medical scrolls written over a period of 800 years or more. The most famous of these scrolls are the Smith and Ebers papyri, which date back to 1650 B.C. and 1550 B.C., respectively. The Smith papyrus, however, is believed by some scholars to be a copy of a much older scroll written approximately 3000 B.C. It appears that physicians were common in ancient Egypt and, medically speaking, they were somewhat more sophisticated than the Mesopotamians. From the Smith and Ebers papyri, for example, we learned that the Egyptians may have been the first people to use wooden splints for fractures. The papyri also revealed the Egyptians as adept in at least two of the three healing gestures: (1) the preparation of plasters and (2) the application of bandages. The Egyptians may have been the first people to use adhesive bandages and were almost certainly the first people to apply honey to wounds.

Statue of Imhotep (circa 2600 B.C.), who Sir William Osler called "the first figure of a physician to stand out clearly from the mists of antiquity." Imhotep was granted full status as a god in 500 B.C. and was later adopted by the Greeks, who named him "Asklepios."

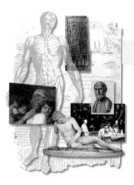

The Egyptians also emphasized careful examination of the wound. Most of the treatment regimens translated from the medical papyri begin with palpation of the wound. Take, for example, this description from the Smith papyrus:

"If thou examinest a man having a gaping wound in his head, penetrating to the bone, splitting his skull, thou shouldst palpate his wound. Shouldst thou find something disturbing therein under thy fingers..."

Palpating the wound, or the "laying of hands" upon the wound, appears in some contexts to have ritualistic implications. It is also clear, however, from the example above that the Egyptian physician, or "swnw," was well aware of the importance of examining the wound and that the course of treatment was influenced by the results of the examination. Thus, we see perhaps the first example of the clinical decision-making process guided by "nonritualistic" examination of the patient.

The writings in the Smith papyrus provide a remarkable example of the efficiency with which the "swnw" contended with wounds. Each case description (there were 48 in the Smith papyrus alone) consisted of what we would call an examination, a diagnosis, and a treatment. After examining the wound, the "swnw" would place it in one of three categories depending on the severity of the injury:

1 an ailment that he would treat

2 an ailment with which he would contend

3 an ailment not to be treated

This is the first written evidence of medical triage. The descriptions contained in the Smith papyrus suggest that wounds were diagnosed and treated according to the severity of the problem.

Egyptian Wound Dressings

Honey, grease, and lint were the main components of the most common plaster used by the Egyptians. The Egyptians apparently had great confidence in this mixture, as it is recommended for the treatment of almost all types of external wounds. Lint, most likely made from vegetable fiber, probably aided drainage of the wound; grease and honey may have protected the wound from infection.

Grease made from animal fat may have provided a barrier to bacteria, while honey appears to be an effective antibacterial agent and is bacteriostatic for gram-positive organisms. The antibacterial properties of honey are the result of several factors. First, honey is extremely hypertonic and therefore kills bacteria by osmotic shrinkage

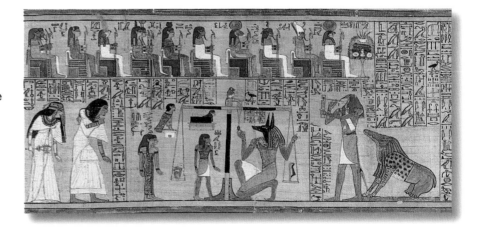

Scene from the Egyptian Book of the Dead (circa 1250 B.C.) showing Anubis weighing a supplicant's heart on scales symbolizing truth.

while also drawing fluid from the wound. Second, it contains glucose oxidase, which produces hydrogen peroxide, a mild antibacterial agent. Finally, honey contains galangine, which is used today as a food preservative. The mixture of grease and honey may also have prevented bandages from sticking to the wound much the same as oil does. Honey proved to be so valuable in promoting wound healing that the practice of smearing honey on wounds lasted for thousands of years and is still used by

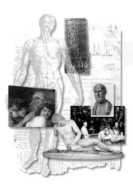

some cultures. The use of honey (but not grease) was adopted by the Greeks, who were heavily influenced by Egyptian culture. Honey was also used for wound care in India long before the time of Christ, demonstrating that separate medical cultures empirically arrived at the same approach to successful therapy.

The painting of body parts had immense ritualistic meaning for Egyptians, much as it does for Native Americans. In Egypt, however, wounds were painted as well. To prepare the colorful paints, they often used mineral ores, the color of the paint depending on the mineral contained in the ore. Since wounds are associated with death, it seems natural that the Egyptians would paint wounds with green paint (called "wadj"), as the color green was symbolic of life—not surprising for a culture surrounded on either side by deserts. But, it is quite possible that aside from the psychological solace provided to the patient, painting the wound provided a direct benefit to wound healing. Each of the minerals used to make green paint contains copper, which is toxic to bacteria and may have helped decrease bacterial counts in infected wounds. Two of the more common ores used to make green pigment were malachite (copper carbonate) and chrysocolla (copper silicate).

Image of the god Osiris from the opening scene of the Book of the Dead of Khai (circa 1540 B.C.).

The art of preventing decomposition (which is largely the result of bacteria) by embalming may have contributed to early advances in controlling infection.

Egyptian Bandages: The "awy"

Perhaps more than any other ancient civilization, the Egyptians excelled in bandaging—what they called the "awy." When most people think of ancient Egypt, they think of pyramids and mummies. In Egypt, the bandaging of the dead was part of a highly religious ceremony during which the nobility were prepared for eternal life. The art of wrapping the bodies of the dead probably influenced the bandaging of wounds, at least to some extent. For example, adhesive bandages for wounds were prepared by dipping them in various gums and resins. These resins were also commonly used as preservatives by embalmers. Natural resins are clear, semisolid, viscous substances, such as amber, produced by numerous plants and shrubs. The most common resins used in Egypt were myrrh and frankincense. Although myrrh was not native to Egypt and had to be imported from extreme east Africa and lower Arabia, it was used extensively in wound healing, indicating the confidence that the "swnw" had in this resin. Why resins were used for wounds is not clear, but Majno suggests three reasons. First, the Egyptians may have reasoned that since sap or resin exudes from wounded trees, it may be beneficial to treat wounded humans.

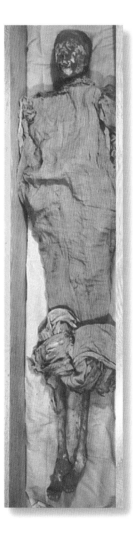

Mummified remains of Pharaoh Siphtah (circa 1300 B.C.)

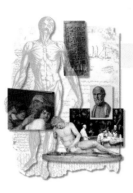

Second, resins are known for their fragrance (they were also used in perfumes and incense), and thus they may be useful in treating malodorous (ie, infected) wounds. Third, resins are resistant to decay, and therefore it was hoped that they would transfer this property to the wound.

It seems likely that adhesive bandages were used in ancient Egypt for much the same reasons they are used today: to hold the margins of the wound together, to protect the wound from re-injury, and in some cases to hold the dressing in place. The Egyptians may also have stitched wounds (what they called the "ydr"), and here again, the art of managing wounds in the living may have been influenced by the art of preparing the bodies of the dead, for the oldest known stitches are preserved on a mummy dating back to circa 1100 B.C. Adhesive bandages, like modern skin tapes, appeared to be the preferred method of closing wounds. The Egyptians were also known to use meat to close wounds, similar to the way allografts or pig skin are used today.

....

The process of mummification involved extensive and often elaborate bandaging. The process began with the removal of the internal organs, from which the Egyptians may have gained some rudimentary knowledge of human anatomy.

The Good Wound and the Bad Wound

The Egyptians may have also been the first to distinguish between infected, what they called "bad" or "diseased" wounds, and uninfected, or "good," wounds (although the concept of infection as such would not be developed for several millennia). They even went so far as to give wounds different names depending on the degree of "badness." For example, "wbnw" signified what we would call an uninfected, or sterile, wound; whereas "bnwt," which was described as "brother of blood, friend of pus, father of the jackal," probably referred to a diseased, or infected, wound.

The Egyptians, nevertheless, recognized the different healing potential of these two types of wounds. Infected wounds were characterized by a "whirl of inflammation," by the feverish state of the patient, and by the tendency of the wound to "throw pus" and were treated differently from "good" wounds. Whereas uninfected wounds were treated according to the three healing gestures, infected wounds were left open and stimulated to produce pus. Animal fat or rotted meat was placed on the wound as a means to this end. The production of pus was considered beneficial to healing "sick" (ie, infected) wounds, although the scientific basis for this concept would not emerge for several millennia.

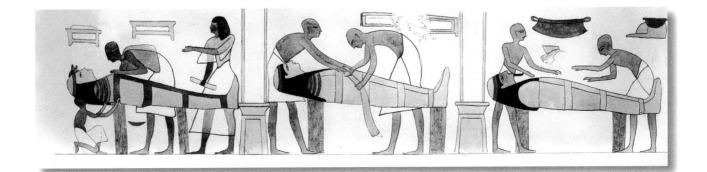

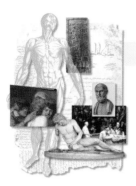

THE GREEK TRADITION

" ...yet the physician must explore thy wound, and with his balsams soothe the bitter pain. "

- Homer, the Iliad

Bust of the Greek physician Hippocrates. Much of what is known about Greek medicine comes to us from his collection of medical writings (The Hippocratic Collection).

Leaving behind a vast historic record, the Egyptians had an immense influence on the Greeks and the Romans, and hence on the Western world. Greek medicine, however, should be considered an extension, rather than a mere reflection, of Egyptian medicine. The Greeks took what they considered as the best Egyptian medicine had to offer and, in many respects, improved upon it; in some cases, their contributions were original.

Much of what is known about Greek medicine comes to us from the medical writings of Hippocrates (The Hippocratic Collection). The use of wine and vinegar (acetic acid) to treat wounds, for example, was a major contribution to wound healing. The Greeks used wine and vinegar to wash the wound, they diluted many of their plasters in it, and they even soaked bandages in it. Although these methods were used for thousands of years, the scientific basis for their benefits remained unknown for many centuries. We now know that acetic acid is an effective antimicrobial agent, particularly against pseudomonads.

The list of Greek "firsts" in medicine is impressive. In addition to being the first to use wine to treat wounds, they may also have been the first to recognize the danger of gangrene associated with the use of tourniquets or ligatures and recommended that they not be left on too long. In this respect, the Greeks appeared to have a better grasp of the concept of hemostasis than previous civilizations. They also recommended applying cold water around the wound to stop bleeding.

The Greeks stressed the importance of cleanliness. Not only did they recommend washing the wound with clean water (often boiled first), vinegar, and wine, but they also had a host of recommendations as to the appearance, cleanliness, and demeanor of the physician (the "iatros"), even going so far as to describe how the physician should stand while treating his patients.

For the most part, wound dressings in ancient Greece were similar to those used in Egypt and Mesopotamia; they consisted of extracts of various plants, oils, resins (myrrh and frankincense, again) and inorganic salts: what the Greeks called "a drug for fresh wounds."

"Fresh" Versus "Nonhealing" Wounds

The Greeks may have been the first to distinguish between "fresh" and "nonhealing" wounds. This is a much more subtle distinction than the one made by the Egyptians (ie, infected versus uninfected wounds). We are only now beginning to understand what distinguishes an acute wound from a nonhealing (ie, chronic) wound. The Greeks were also familiar with the concept of cutaneous ulcers. They understood the value of relieving pressure at the ulcer site and recommended that the patient stay off his or her feet. Otherwise, they believed the ulcer would heal more slowly. In fact, The Hippocratic Collection contains an elegant description of a woman who suffered from a venous ulcer as a result of varicose veins. It is apparent from the description that the Greeks were aware that skin ulcers were slow to heal, as indicated by this excerpt from The Hippocratic Collection:

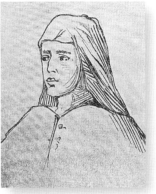

Herophilus (born circa 335 B.C.), the grandson of Aristotle and founder of the school of anatomy in Alexandria, helped provide an anatomical foundation for the study of medicine.

> *For an obstinate ulcer, sweet wine and alot of patience should be enough...*

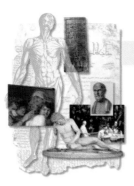

The Alexandrian School

During the Hippocratic Era, the study of anatomy was not approached as an observational science. Instead, the early Greeks preferred to visualize the structure of the body using the "mind's eye." Fortunately, this was not the case in Alexandria, where the study of anatomy was pioneered.

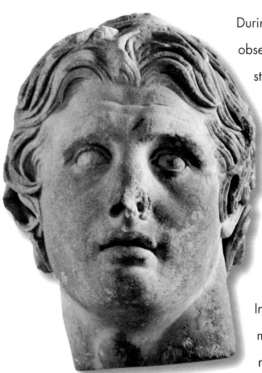

Alexandria was founded by Alexander the Great in 332 B.C. The city was built on the western delta of the Nile and was home of the Great Library, which was said to contain as many as 750,000 volumes, including the complete works of Alexander's teacher, Aristotle. The library, along with all its contents, was later destroyed in part by Julius Caesar, then by Christian zealots over the centuries. In addition to the Great Library, Alexandria was home of one of the first museums, which was actually a scientific institute. Here, scholars from many different disciplines, including medicine, studied and taught. The major field of medical research at the Alexandrian Museum was anatomy—a discipline that was unknown to the Hippocratics. In Alexandria, dissection of animals and cadavers and vivisection of animals, and even humans, were performed. Two of its most famous alumni were its founder, Herophilus (called the Father of Anatomy), who was also the grandson of Aristotle, and Erasistratus. Interestingly, Erasistratus did not condone the practice of bloodletting, which was widely practiced at that time. As a result, he earned the enmity of another famous Greek physician, Galen, whose influence would dominate medicine for centuries.

Marble head of Alexander the Great, found in Pergamon. He founded the city of Alexandria on the banks of the Nile, which became the center of medical learning in the Hellenic world.

"*...it is better for the patient to drown in his own blood than to be bled.*"
- Erasistratus

The art of bloodletting was later refined in the 14th century by the introduction of leeches to bleed patients. As many as 3,000,000 leeches per year were used in France alone during the 14th century. By the early 19th century, the annual demand for leeches had risen to approximately 20,000,000. Some historians have suggested that the deaths of Mozart and George Washington were hastened by frequent bloodlettings.

Next to pioneering the study of anatomy, perhaps the greatest contribution of Alexandrian medicine to wound healing was the technique of ligating vessels to stop bleeding. Before the founding of the Alexandrian school, hemostasis was achieved by cautery—a technique developed by the Egyptians and re-introduced by the Arabs during the Dark Ages. The technique of ligating blood vessels had two important clinical consequences: (1) it led to advances in surgery and (2) it encouraged the practice of bloodletting because physicians were no longer overly worried about uncontrolled bleeding resulting from bloodletting. Physicians believed that if a person died during a bloodletting at least he died "healthy."

Celsus: The Four Cardinal Signs of Inflammation

Roman medicine borrowed much from the Greeks. In fact, during the early years of the Roman Empire, most of the physicians in Rome were Greek. Perhaps the most lasting contribution of Rome to medicine was made by Celsus. Aurelius Cornelius Celsus may not have been a physician himself, but he wrote an eight-volume compendium of medicine (*De Medicina*) that was to become one of the most influential medical texts ever written. It contained an early description of the "four cardinal signs of inflammation," which are: rubor, tumor, calor et dolor (redness, swelling, heat, and pain). *De Medicina* vanished soon after it was published and did not resurface until 1426. Fifty years after its reappearance, it was to be among the first medical texts printed on the newly invented printing press.

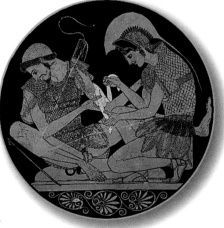

This battlefield scene, from the bowl of Sosias (circa 50 B.C.) shows Achilles bandaging the wounds of Patroclus.

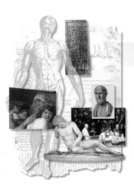

The Four Bodily Humors

The Greeks advanced the study of medicine in general and wound healing in particular. The method of dousing wounds with wine was a step forward because of the antiseptic properties of wine. Not all the practices condoned by the Greeks, however, were beneficial. As for medical theory, the Greeks believed that all diseases resulted from an imbalance in the four bodily "humors" (blood, phlegm, yellow bile, and black bile). The theory of bodily humors would dominate medicine for centuries.

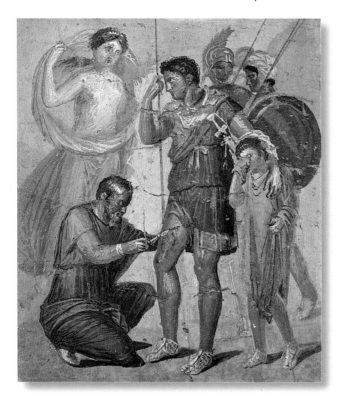

The Hippocratic tradition held that all diseases (wounds at that time were considered diseases) could be cured by restoring the humoral balance or eliminating the bad humor either by bleeding the patient or by encouraging suppuration (formation of pus), or frequently, both. A substantial part of medicine at that time was devoted to the practice of bloodletting—a practice that goes back to ancient times. The Egyptians, for example, practiced bloodletting, but it was not until the time of Hippocrates that it achieved the status as a remedy for all ills. Bloodletting was performed for every illness, from consumption to melancholia. Its practice was further encouraged by another famous physician, Galen, who attempted to provide a scientific foundation for its practice.

A 1st century fresco entitled "Aeneas Receiving Treatment for a Wound." The physician, Iapyx, is shown removing an arrowhead with forceps.

Galen

After Hippocrates, Galen may have been the most influential physician in
history. He was born in Pergamon circa 130 A.D. and received his medical
training in Smyrna, Corinth, and Alexandria. Shortly after, he returned to
Pergamon as a physician to gladiators, where he was exposed to many
types of traumatic wounds. Later, he moved to Rome and served as court
physician to Emperor Marcus Aurelius, but he fell from favor with later
emperors. He died circa 200 A.D., probably in exile. Although his views
on medicine were, for the most part, Hippocratic, in one respect he departed
from the Hippocratic tradition. He practiced dissection, no doubt as a result
of the training he received in many cities, including Alexandria. Thus, his
lasting contributions were mainly in the area of anatomy.

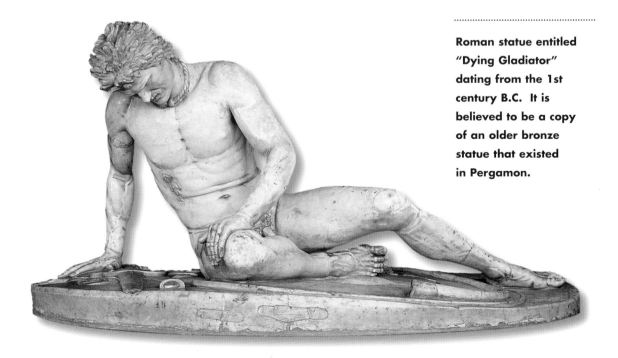

**Roman statue entitled
"Dying Gladiator"
dating from the 1st
century B.C. It is
believed to be a copy
of an older bronze
statue that existed
in Pergamon.**

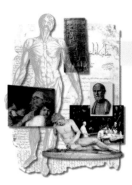

After the fall of Rome, the Arabs, who were strongly influenced by Galen and Hippocrates, also added further "refinements" to the art of bloodletting by defining the conditions under which it should be performed. For example, Arabic physicians prohibited bloodletting during a full moon, during certain seasons, and when the wind was from the South. Usually it was performed by a barber/surgeon working under the supervision of the physician. At the time of Galen and throughout most of the Dark and Middle Ages, surgery was not considered a distinct branch of medicine.

Since the sick were considered unclean, and disease was considered a punishment for sins, Jewish, Arab, and Christian physicians would rarely practice surgery. Instead, it was performed by barbers, who were not nearly as well educated as physicians. The barber/surgeon lasted through the Middle Ages, and it was not until the 18th century that surgery began to be considered as a distinct, and respected, branch of medicine.

Illustration from a mid-13th century manuscript showing a physician bandaging a wound after applying an ointment made from cream, honey, and herbs.

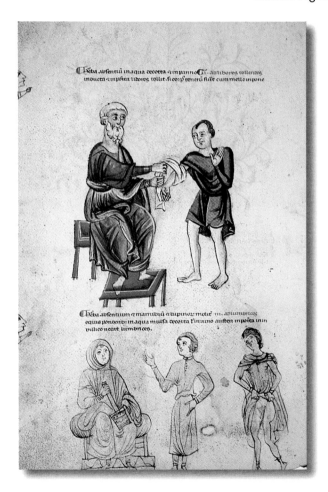

MEDIEVAL MEDICINE

There were few advancements in wound healing made during the Middle Ages. In some respects, due to the decline of Greek influence in Europe, wound care practice actually regressed. Although the Greek tradition in wound healing was preserved through the Middle Ages by monks and by Jewish physicians, who were, along with the Arabs, considered the most knowledgeable physicians in Europe, most of the original medical writings of the Greeks and Romans were lost after the fall of Rome. Fortunately, many medical texts had been translated into Arabic by Arabic physicians, such as Avicenna, during the Middle Ages. As a result, most of those writings now found in Greek and Latin are retranslations from Arabic. These texts would almost certainly have been lost forever had it not been for Arabic scholars.

The most popular treatment for wounds, or any disease for that matter, continued to be bloodletting; the causes of infection remained a complete mystery; honey was smeared on wounds, along with other much less pleasant substances, such as dove's dung (a favorite of Galen's); and bandages were still soaked in wine and vinegar. With the exception of a brief spark that appeared during the 12th century and would resurface several hundred years later, progress in wound healing appeared to be at a complete standstill.

A page from an Arabic translation of Galen (11th century) bearing the signature of Avicenna.

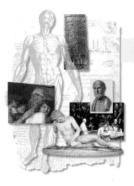

A Brief Spark: Theodoric and the Salernitan School

Legend has it that the school of medicine in Salerno, Italy was founded in the 10th century by an Arab, a Jewish rabbi, a Greek, and an unknown native of Salerno. During the Middle Ages, the Salernitan School was the center of medical learning. Two of its most famous graduates were Hugo of Lucco and his pupil Theodoric of Bologna (also called Theodoric of Cervia). Theodoric (Teodorico Borgognoni), who some scholars say was Hugo's son, was born in 1205 and became a Dominican friar in 1226. He was trained by Hugo and eventually taught at the University of Bologna. Theodoric was by most accounts an excellent and scholarly physician. Although the theory of laudable pus was universally accepted as one of the principles of wound healing, Theodoric, like Hippocrates before him, believed that pus was not necessary for healing of all types of wounds. However, whereas Hippocrates believed that the production of pus had no positive effects on wound healing, Theodoric held that the production of pus was detrimental to, and actually delayed, healing of some types of wounds. Instead, he was a proponent of healing *per primum*, or healing by primary intent (a phrase attributed to one of his students, Henri de Mondeville) and promoted a standardized method of wound healing that included cleaning the wound with acetic acid, removing dead tissue by debridement, closing the wound with stitches, and applying a protective bandage.

Guy de Chauliac is regarded as one of the most influential French surgeons despite his rejection of Theodoric's teachings. His method of wound management was, overall, an improvement over older methods. It consisted of five principles:

1) removing foreign matter,

2) re-approximating the separated parts,

3) preserving the parts in their original form,

4) preserving and conserving the substance, and

5) correcting complications.

Unfortunately, Theodoric's techniques were abandoned after the death of his pupil, the French surgeon Henri de Mondeville, and did not resurface for 700 years. Although this is not entirely understood, several reasons for the failure of Theodoric's theories have been suggested. One reason may be that Mondeville's manuscript on surgery, which presumably incorporated a great deal of Theodoric's methods, was never completed. Perhaps more importantly, Theodoric's teachings were discredited, mainly by another famous French surgeon, Guy de Chauliac, who accused him of plagiarism. The surgeon Eldridge Campbell, who served as surgical consultant in the Mediterranean theatre during World War II, has suggested that Mondeville's irreverent personality may have been the primary reason for the rejection of his theories. In any case, the influence of the Salernitan School gradually faded, and shortly after, under the guidance of Guy de Chauliac, France became the center of medical training in Europe. The first medical school in France, and one of the oldest in Europe, was established at Montpelier in the 10th century.

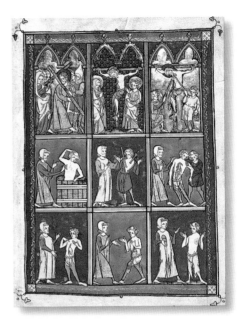

Page from a 13th century French translation of Roger of Salerno's Chirurgia, showing different methods of treating wounds. The word "surgery" is believed to be derived from "chirurgia."

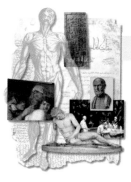

RENAISSANCE: THE REBIRTH OF MEDICINE

It was after the end of the Middle Ages and during the Renaissance that the art of wound healing began once again to make progress. The Hippocratic tradition, reinforced by the writings of Galen, continued to dominate medicine. Surgery, as we know it, was still not considered part of medicine proper. Although the influence of the church over medicine began to fade and medicine took on a more secular flavor, these trends would likely have continued had it not been for the efforts of two of Europe's most revered physicians: Ambroise Paré and Andreas Vesalius.

Anatomy and Surgery Come of Age

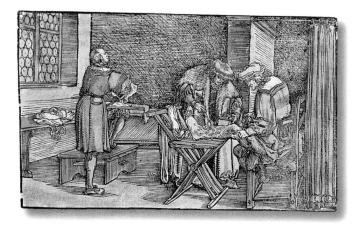

Hospital treatment of a leg ulcer during the Middle Ages. Illustration from "Der Grossen Wundarztney," by Paracelsus.

Considered the father of modern anatomy, Andreas Vesalius (1514–1564) was a Flemish physician who pioneered the dissection of human cadavers. His careful descriptions of the human structure helped establish anatomy as a modern observational science. In 1543, the same year that Copernicus published his *De Revolutionibus Orbium Coelestrium* (On the Revolution of the Celestial Spheres), Vesalius published the beautifully illustrated *De Humani Corporis Fabrica* (On the Fabric of the Human Body). Vesalius taught at the University of Padua, and afterwards he was physician to the Holy Roman Emperor Charles V and to Philip II, King of Spain. In part through his influence, northern Italy became the center for the study of medicine in general, and human anatomy in particular, during the 16th century.

Ambroise Paré (1510–1590), considered the father of surgery, was the son of a French cabinet maker. He helped establish surgery as a separate and indispensable branch of medicine. In 1533, Paré became an apprentice barber in Paris, where he studied anatomy and surgery. In 1537, he became an army surgeon, eventually rising to the rank of surgeon for King Henry II in 1552. When Paré began his career as an army surgeon, the standard method for managing gunshot wounds was to treat them with hot oil and cautery. The technique of ligating bleeding vessels, which had been developed by Greek and Egyptian physicians at the Alexandrian school, had been abandoned during the Dark Ages when the Arabs re-introduced the practice of cautery. During a particularly bloody battle, Paré ran out of hot oil and, forced to find an alternative, he used a mixture of turpentine, rose oil, and egg whites to treat the wounds of soldiers. The next morning, he hurried to the battlefield to inspect the soldiers' wounds, fearing that his substitute treatment may have caused harm to his patients. In his own words:

> *I could not sleep that night, for I was troubled in mind, and the dressing of the precedent day, (which I judged unfit) troubled my thoughts; and I feared that the next day would find them dead by the poison of the wound, whom I had not dressed by the scalding oil. Therefore I rose early in the morning. I visited my patients and beyond expectation, I found such as I had dressed with the digestive only, free from vehemence of pain to have good rest, and that their wounds were not inflamed, not tumifyed; but on the contrary the others that were burnt with the scalding oil were feverish, tormented with much pain, and the parts about their wounds were swollen.*

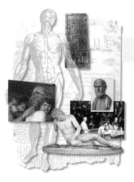

From then on, he vowed never to treat injuries with hot oil. His contribution to general surgery includes the re-introduction of ligatures to control bleeding. He also devised artificial limbs, improved the treatment of fractures, and developed several surgical and orthopedic devices.

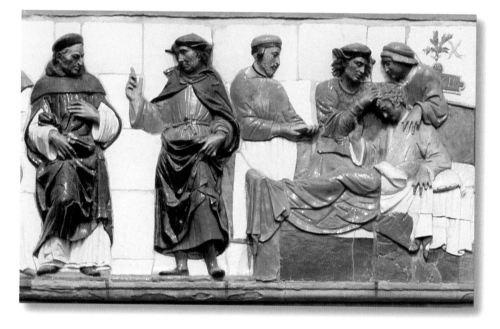

Portion of a 16th century frieze called "Visiting the Sick," by Giovanni Della Robbia.

Paré and Vesalius were contemporaries, and even though one specialized in surgery and the other in anatomy, they were considered two of the brightest stars in the field of medicine during the 16th century, which indicates how important these fields were becoming in the practice of medicine. Thus, when King Henry II was wounded in the head with a lance during a tournament, both Paré and Vesalius were summoned. Together, the two physicians dissected the heads of four cadavers trying to determine the nature and extent of the king's injuries. Ultimately they failed and the king died, but as Phillip Rhodes points out: "this may have been one of the earliest recourses to the laboratory to solve a pressing clinical problem." It is also an early example of the close association these two fields would have in the future.

ENLIGHTENMENT: THE AGE OF ANTISEPSIS

Until the 18th century, the history of medicine was dominated by physicians and philosophers. All that was about to change. During the Renaissance, mysticism and blind faith slowly gave way to reason and logic. Scientists, some with little or no medical training, began to exert an influence on wound healing. This trend continued during the Enlightenment.

Elucidating the mechanisms of infection during the 18th and 19th centuries was among the greatest advancements contributing to the understanding of wound healing. Each of the three ancient healing gestures (interventions) can be viewed as a variation on the theme of controlling bacterial infection. Paradoxically, those who practiced wound healing were operating under contradictory assumptions: they were concerned with preventing infection (even if they were unaware of its mechanisms) while simultaneously introducing substances into the wound that would cause infection and induce the formation of pus.

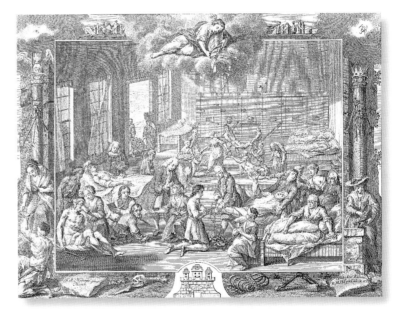

1746 engraving entitled "The Plague Ward," showing a doctor amputating a patient's leg (center).

The English surgeon John Hunter (1728–1793), considered by many to be the founder of modern surgery, was one of the dominant personalities in medicine during the 1700s. Before him, surgery was considered a subordinate branch of medicine. John Hunter made surgery a science and raised it to a status equal to that of clinical medicine. His *Treatise on the Blood, Inflammation and Gun-shot Wounds*, published in 1794, was considered the most important step in understanding the process of inflammation since Celsus described the "four cardinal signs."

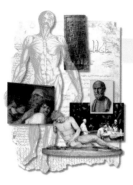

Progress in the Early 19th Century

In the 19th century, wound healing came into its own. It was in this century that the cause of infection, as well as its prevention, were beginning to be elucidated, and progress was made toward understanding the cellular processes that contribute to inflammation. These advances were, as one can imagine, not the work of a single person but the culmination of the work of many people—all working at about the same time.

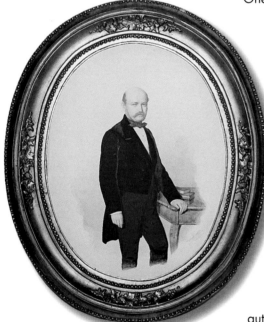

Ignatz Philipp Semmelweis, 1818–1865.

....

One of the most tragic, yet influential, figures in the history of medicine is Ignatz Philipp Semmelweis. He was born in Hungary in 1818, studied medicine in Hungary and Vienna, and in 1846 was appointed Assistant in the First Obstetric Clinic of the famous Allgemeines Krankenhaus in Vienna. At that time, approximately 3 of every 20 women who gave birth died from puerperal (childbed) fever. In 1843, the American physician/writer Oliver Wendell Holmes suggested that puerperal fever is a contagious septicemia transmitted to new mothers from infected patients by obstetricians. His idea met with ridicule, and he did not pursue his theory. When one of Semmelweis' professors at the school died following a wound he received during a postmortem dissection, Semmelweis noted at the autopsy that his symptoms were similar to those of women who had died of puerperal fever. He also observed that the incidence of puerperal fever was lower in the ward attended by midwives compared with that of the ward attended by students. These two observations led him to speculate, as Holmes did, that puerperal fever resulted from the introduction of some contagion carried by the students from the postmortem dissection room to the obstetrics ward, where students would seldom wash their hands before examining the women or delivering a child. Therefore, he introduced the practice of scrubbing one's hands with soap and water, then rinsing them in a hypochlorite solution before examining a patient.

One of the great figures in the 19th century was Rudolph Virchow (1821-1902). Virchow, considered the founder of modern cellular pathology, was well respected in every field he chose to study, whether it was medicine, science, politics, philosophy, or anthropology. In 1858, he published Cellular Pathology, *which remained for many decades as the standard textbook of pathology. His doctrine of* omnis cellula e cellula *("where a cell arises, there a cell must have previously existed") set the stage for Pasteur and Lister.*

The incidence of puerperal fever dropped from 15% to 1% in both wards, but Semmelweis' method was so unorthodox, and met with such fierce opposition, that he was forced to leave Vienna and eventually came to practice at a small hospital in Budapest. There, he continued his struggle to introduce antiseptic practices, meeting with much the same success as he had previously in Vienna (within 2 years, the incidence of puerperal fever dropped to less than 1%), but his methods continued to be ignored, and he was often treated with open hostility by his colleagues within the medical profession. In 1865, after a lifelong struggle against jealous colleagues, according to one account, Semmelweis died in a Vienna insane asylum from an infected wound.

Joseph Lister and the Antiseptic Technique

We have come to know of the contributions of Semmelweis in the field of antisepsis in part due to another giant in the struggle against infection— Joseph Lister. It is a tribute to Lister that he gave credit where it was due by acknowledging Semmelweis' work in the field. Joseph Lister was born in England in 1827, received his Bachelor of Arts from the University of London in 1847 and his Bachelor of Medicine in 1852. At that time, as many as 80% of wounds became gangrenous. Amputation was the most common procedure performed by surgeons, and approximately 40% of patients died

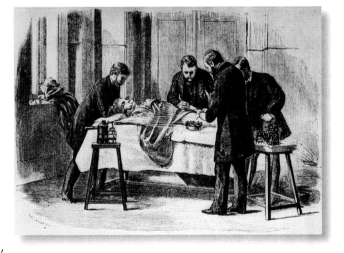

"Antiseptic Surgery," by W. Watson, showing the use of carbolic spray first promoted by Lister.

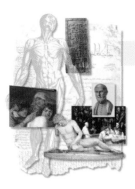

from infection—in some hospitals the mortality rate was as high as 90%. Paradoxically, the mortality rate was much lower in country practices, so much so that patients came to dread hospitalization. Death from infection contracted while hospitalized came to be known as "hospitalism," and in some places, existing hospitals were demolished and new ones were prohibited from being built. This is the atmosphere in which Lister came to practice.

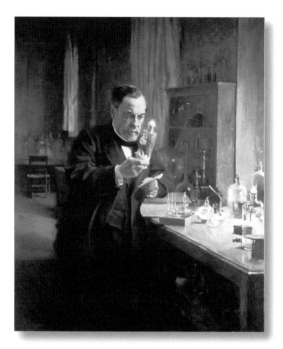

Portrait of Louis Pasteur in his laboratory, by Albert-Gustaf Edelfelt.

Lister was a strong proponent of general cleanliness in the hospital and the frequent use of soap and water. He experimented with several methods of treating wounds, including the "open method" favored by some surgeons, in which the wound was left open and allowed to heal on its own. He also tried the occlusion method used by his colleagues in Edinburgh, in which the wound was sealed with collodion. Neither approach worked. He decided that in order to solve the problem of suppuration, he must first understand its nature. Realizing that "foul discharges from sores were the predisposing cause" of gangrene, Lister set about finding the causative agent. Thus, he was led naturally to the work of Pasteur.

A chemist by training, Louis Pasteur (1822–1895) was appointed director of scientific studies at the Ecole Normale in 1857, where he began his studies on the process of fermentation. The existence of microorganisms had already been proven with the aid of Leeuwenhoek's microscope. Pasteur proved conclusively that bacteria were responsible for the process of fermentation and putrefaction. He then set about disproving the theory of spontaneous generation, which was widely believed at that time, and in 1863 Pasteur invented the process that still bears his name: pasteurization.

Pasteur's work was brought to the attention of Lister in 1860, and it immediately suggested to him that germs are the causative agents in infection. Since bacteria did not spontaneously generate, as Pasteur had proved, it seemed reasonable that they were introduced into wounds from some foreign source, as Holmes and Semmelweis had believed. So, Lister set about developing his antiseptic technique. He continued to advocate frequent washing with soap and water and general cleanliness in the clinic, but most of his energy was spent in search of ways to kill bacteria. Pasteur had previously shown that heat kills organisms. Lister was aware that germs can also be killed by certain chemicals. He decided the chemical approach was the most practical:

It occurred to me that decomposition in the injured part might be avoided without excluding air by applying as a dressing some material capable of destroying the life of the floating particles.

Lister experimented with many different chemicals in his search to find an effective antiseptic before he finally settled on carbolic acid, or phenol. He not only dressed wounds with lint soaked in carbolic acid, he also soaked surgical instruments and ligatures in it prior to surgery, and even sprayed the operating arena with a carbolic acid spray during surgical procedures. The results were dramatic, and even though his practices met with skepticism in the medical world initially, his results were so impressive that within a few years, the antiseptic technique came to be standard operating procedure in Europe, followed soon after by the aseptic technique. It was not possible for him to know at that time that carbolic acid is actually toxic to the hosts' cells, and therefore impedes healing, despite its ability to control infection. Nevertheless, its use was a major advance in the field of wound healing. Semmelweis, Virchow, Pasteur, Lister, and a host of others working, for the most part, during the middle of the 19th century established a scientific basis for the management of wounds.

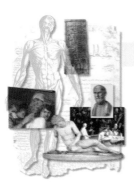

Medicine in America

In the United States, Lister's method was adopted slowly. Even as late as the 1880s, American physicians regarded aseptic technique with skepticism. However, Lister's ideas eventually caught on. In 1897, Fred Kilmer (father of the poet Joyce Kilmer) published *Asepsis Secundum Artem* (Following the Art of Asepsis), which was considered a classic on the subject of sterility in wound healing.

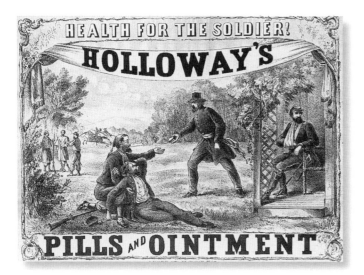

1863 advertisement for Holloway's Pills and Ointment. At that time, there were few regulations regarding the production and use of drugs.

Medical practice in America generally lagged behind European medicine, particularly during the Colonial period. For the most part, medicine was practiced by men with little, if any, formal training. Those few physicians who practiced in America were educated in Europe, mainly in Edinburgh, Paris, and later Germany. As the country grew and prospered, however, the medical tradition took root. Philadelphia, along with Boston and New York, became the centers of medical training in America. The first hospital was established in Philadelphia in 1752. Thirteen years later, John Morgan and William Shippen established the first medical school at what is now the University of Pennsylvania. In 1850, the first fully approved, legal women's medical school in the world, The Female Medical College of Pennsylvania (later called the Women's Medical College of Pennsylvania), was established. The most influential physicians, nevertheless, continued to be trained in Europe.

The description of the septic death of General "Stonewall" Jackson is a dramatic example of the injured dignitary whose amputation was delayed because of his famous name.

During the American Civil War, few physicians were aware of the work of Pasteur and Lister. However, civil war surgeons recognized that amputation of a missile-wounded extremity within hours following injury often prevented septic death. Like Hunter before them, they knew that these large open wounds would heal by contraction if kept clean and open.

During the early part of the 19th century, when the country was still growing and there were few legal restrictions governing medical training, more than 400 medical schools existed. Most of these schools were little more than "diploma mills." Few offered more than a short course or two in medical training. The low standards of most of these schools contributed to the generally low quality of medical education in the United States. The outbreak of the American Civil War further exacerbated the situation, as many of the South's medical centers were destroyed or dissolved during the war. After the Civil War, medical education in America began to recover, partly through the efforts of the American Medical Association, which was established in 1847. The diploma mills continued to proliferate, however, until Simon Flexner's report from the Rockefeller Institute in 1910 exposed their shortcomings and placed medical education in proper academic settings.

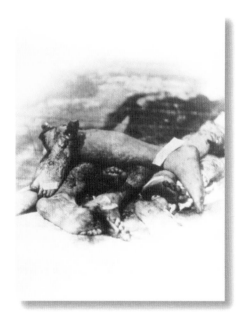

Civil War era wounds resulted in frequent lower extremity amputations as evidenced by this photograph of a pile of legs.

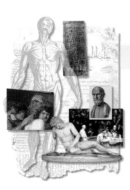

WOUND HEALING IN THE 20TH CENTURY

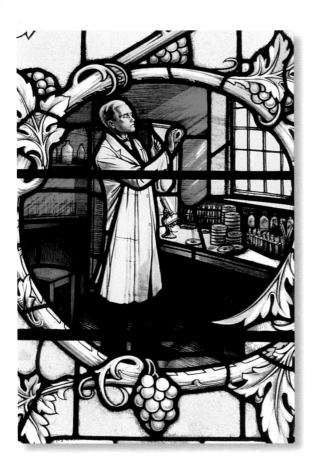

Stained glass window in St. James Church in London depicting Sir Alexander Fleming at work in his laboratory. Fleming won the Nobel Prize for his serendipitous discovery of the antibiotic properties of penicillin in 1928.

Wound healing research made rapid progress following the discovery of the nature and causes of infection. Antiseptic technique, in which the growth of infectious agents is slowed or prevented, was followed shortly by aseptic technique, in which a sterile environment (ie, one free of infectious agents) is achieved. Metallic antiseptics, such as mercuric bichloride, were introduced late in the 19th century. In the early part of the 20th century, the use of antiseptics was followed by much wider use of Erlich's chemotherapies, such as sulfonamides in the 1930s, and shortly after by the introduction of antibiotics such as penicillin. Hypochlorite solution, used to combat puerperal fever by Semmelweis, was re-introduced in the early 1900s. A modified hypochlorite solution was used in World War I at the suggestion of Henry Dakin, then a pharmacologist at the Rockefeller Institute, when a fellow member of the Institute serving in France, Alexis Carrel, wrote to him for suggestions for improving treatment of the devastatingly filthy trench wounds. This hypochlorite solution became part of the Carrel-Dakin's method, which consisted of cleansing the wound, liberal irrigation with hypochlorite solution, debridement, and suturing when the wound was clean.

With the rediscovery of Theodoric's methods, wound healing had come almost full circle. The importance of adequate debridement to remove nonviable tissue and to control infection was now fully appreciated. Mortality from infection continued to decline. More effective antibiotics, designed to combat specific infectious agents, were discovered or designed.

The Carrel-Dakin's method for treating osteomyelitis was eventually superseded by the closed-plaster method of Trueta, which had been used during the Spanish Civil War and later during World War II. Treuta's method consisted of thorough debridement of the wound and salting with sulfanilamide powder. Debridement was often accomplished by placing maggots under the cast, which was left in place for long periods to immobilize the injured part. In the latter part of World War II, however, the American surgeon Eldridge Campbell developed the technique of thorough debridement followed by primary closure in certain types of wounds. He was surprised to find that this method had been used by the Italians during World War I. His subsequent research into the subject revealed that healing *per primum* (or healing by primary intent) was the very method developed by Theodoric of Bologna at the Salernitan School in the 13th century.

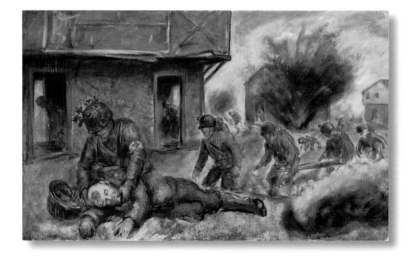

"Medical Training in Texas," by John Steuart Curry (1943).

....

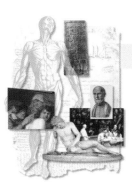

THE ADVENT OF MODERN WOUND HEALING

For most of the 20th century, especially after 1960 and up until the present, research into promoting wound healing has focused for the most part on designing better wound bandages.

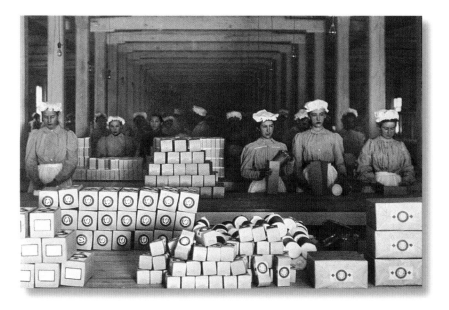

Photograph of workers standing amid boxes of surgical bandages. As a result of technological advances, production of gauze was being counted in "thousands of miles" and bandages in terms of "millions of rolls."

....

The most common bandages were made from wool or linen. Later, in the 19th century, cotton became the material of choice. These materials allow all but the most severe wounds to become dry, especially if they are changed frequently. Although Hippocrates was an advocate of dry healing (he felt this was nearer to the normal condition of the tissue), the concept of wet versus dry wound healing was given little attention. Lister may have been the first person to use bandages specifically to absorb excess drainage, but he also recommended keeping wounds wet with a solution of carbolic acid.

Technological advances such as the cotton gin made possible the large scale production of cotton, which became cheaper to produce than wool—a major factor that contributed to its use as a wound bandage. Because cotton is cheaper than wool, more of it can be used at one time, and dressings can be changed more frequently. Furthermore, with the introduction of sterile cotton gauze at the turn of the century, the demand for this product soared, especially during the wars. Subsequently, manufacturing facilities were built to mass-produce sterile cotton bandages.

Wound Healing at the Cellular Level

In the 19th century, the great cellular pathologist Rudolph Virchow, and his student Julius Cohnheim, laid the foundation for understanding the cellular processes of wound healing. Likewise, Elie Metchnikoff's elegant 1890 treatise *Lessons in Pathology* and later works at the Pasteur Institute laid the foundation for cellular and humoral immunology. With the invention of the electron microscope in the mid-1930s, this process was accelerated. The types of cells involved in wound healing and their functions were now becoming better understood.

In 1962, using an animal model, Winter showed that epithelialization of partial thickness wounds covered with an occlusive dressing was twice as rapid as that of wounds exposed to air. A year later, Hinman and Maibach showed a similar effect in humans. Further study of this phenomenon revealed that removing dry bandages caused secondary trauma, and in the process, the very cells needed to continue wound healing, such as epithelial cells and fibroblasts, were being removed as well.

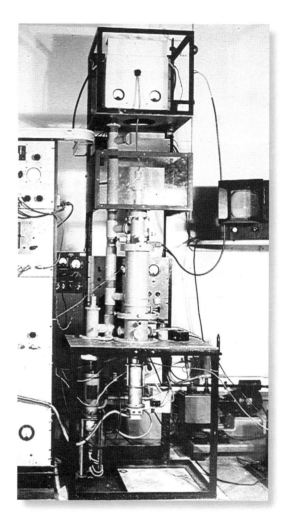

With the invention of the electron microscope in the 1930s, it became possible to study the process of wound healing at the cellular level.

41

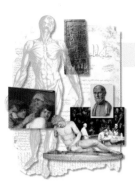

Modern Wound Dressings

The discovery of the benefits of moist wound healing in the 1960s helped improve the management of acute and chronic wounds. There are now more than 2,000 wound care products available, most of which fall into the category of "wound dressings."

Before the cause of infection was understood, the purposes of wound dressings were basically to stop bleeding, protect the wound from re-injury, and to hold the wound edges together. After Lister and Pasteur and until the 1960s, dressings were also used to protect the wound from infection. With the concept of moist wound healing, however, the purposes of dressings expanded considerably. In addition to protecting the wound from infection, we now know that occlusive dressings:

1 *facilitate natural debridement*

2 *minimize inflammation*

3 *reduce pain*

4 *diminish scarring*

Dressings for chronic wounds are now used to:

- Absorb exudate and toxic components
- Provide thermal insulation
- Allow gaseous exchange
- Protect the wound from infection
- Maintain a moist wound environment
- Promote rapid epithelialization
- Relieve pain

The list of types of wound dressings available is impressive. In addition to occlusive dressings, semiocclusive dressings, which are permeable to water vapor and oxygen but impermeable to fluids and bacteria, are now available. The list of available dressings now includes:

- Alginates
- Composites
- Exudate absorbers
- Gauzes
- Foams
- Hydrocolloids
- Hydrogels
- Skin sealants
- Transparent films

Most modern dressings contain materials that are highly absorbent, such as alginates, foam, or carboxymethylcellulose. These dressings are used to absorb exudate while maintaining a moist healing environment. Several dressings are designed to conform to the shape of the wound. Others, such as skin sealants, transparent films, or hydrogels, which simply cover wounds but provide little absorption, are designed for relatively clean, uninfected wounds. These types of dressings must be used cautiously in certain chronic wounds because they do not allow fluid to escape, which may increase the risk of infection.

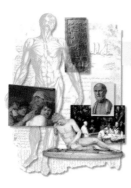

INTO THE FUTURE

In a very broad sense, there have been two schools of philosophic thought regarding the healing process. One held that nature, or God, heals the wound, not the physician. In this view, the physician plays a passive role, his primary concern being to avoid interfering with the natural healing process. This approach is best expressed in the words of Paracelsus, the famous Swiss physician of the 15th century:

"Warily must the surgeon take heed not to remove or interfere with Nature's balsam which healeth wounds. Nature has her own doctor in every limb; wherefore every surgeon should know that it is not he, but Nature, who heals."

The second approach was one in which the physician played a more active role. In this approach, which was common particularly after the cause of infection was understood, the physician took active measures, such as debridement, to heal wounds; or in words attributed to Sir William Osler:

"Empyema requires cold steel, not the folly of a physician."

We now know that the process of wound healing combines these two ideas. Wounds do tend to heal naturally, but the physician can take steps to enhance healing and ensure that no complications, such as infection, occur.

The Next Step in Wound Healing

The wound healing process is now widely recognized as consisting of three distinct, yet overlapping, phases. The first phase, inflammation, which includes coagulation, is characterized by the migration of cells into the wound site. The next phase, the proliferative phase, is characterized by an increase in the number of fibroblasts and a decrease in the number of inflammatory cells at the wound site. The last phase, remodeling, is characterized by maturation of newly produced tissue. These three overlapping phases occur in an orderly fashion, but how is this complex response coordinated? Cellular pathology could not provide the answer. Instead, we must go one step further—to the molecular level.

Physician and novelist Michael Crichton has called biotechnology one of the most powerful technologies ever developed. With this technology, it is possible to modulate the genetic content of a cell, repair genetic defects, and mass-produce proteins such as growth factors, which are normally expressed in such low concentrations that isolating them from their natural source would be impossible. Molecular biological techniques have revolutionized the study of biology and medicine. With these techniques, it may very well become possible to elucidate the mechanisms by which the wound healing response is regulated.

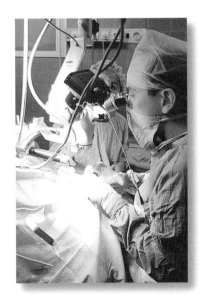

Microsurgical techniques can be used to salvage traumatic amputations and restore function.

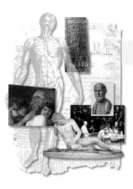

Growth Factors—The Fourth Healing Gesture?

It is now widely believed that the wound healing process is regulated, in part, by the coordinated action of growth factors, such as platelet-derived growth factor (PDGF), transforming growth factor-ß (TGF-ß), and epidermal growth factor (EGF), all of which are synthesized by cells in or near the wound. Identification of the various growth factors involved in wound healing has changed the way wound care is approached. In addition, research into the roles of growth factors has provided clues as to why some wounds heal slowly or not at all—a phenomenon that has puzzled physicians from antiquity. Evidence now suggests that some nonhealing wounds may result from an imbalance in growth factors, protease inhibitors, or metalloproteinases in the wound.

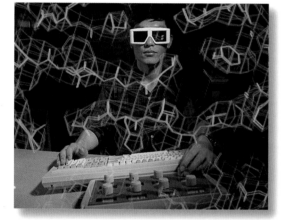

Using modern imaging techniques, it is now possible to construct 3-dimensional models of molecules such as growth factors and other proteins.

Using molecular biological techniques to mass-produce growth factors in genetically engineered yeast or bacteria, it may be possible to promote more efficient healing by directly manipulating the microenvironment of the wound. This new approach is arguably the fourth major advance in wound management.

CONCLUSION

The three healing gestures—washing, dressing, and bandaging—are still practiced today. More than ever, healthcare providers and patients appreciate the importance of cleansing wounds, avoiding infection, and protecting the injury. Countless scientists and physicians have dedicated their lives to understanding and improving upon these three ancient gestures. Now, with the advent of growth factor technology, a new tool in the struggle to promote healing has been added. Will future generations of physicians and healers then study the four healing gestures?

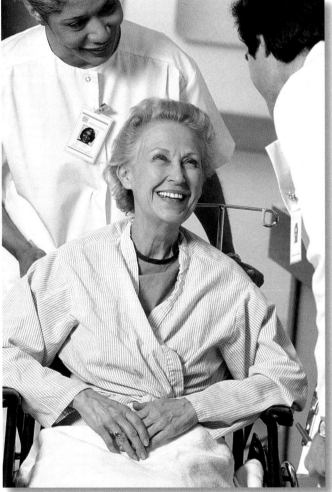

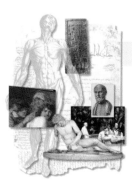

SUGGESTED READINGS

Ackerknecht EH. *A Short History of Medicine*. Baltimore, MD: The Johns Hopkins University Press; 1982.

Bettmann OL. *A Pictorial History of Medicine*. Springfield, IL: Charles C. Thomas; 1956.

Brown H. Wound healing research through the ages. In: Cohen IK, Diegelmann RF, Lindblad WJ, (eds). *Wound Healing: Biochemical and Clinical Aspects*. Philadelphia, PA: W.B. Saunders Company; 1992.

Carmichael AG, Ratzan RM (eds). *Medicine. A Treasury of Art and Literature*. New York, NY: Hugh Lauter Levin Associates, Inc.; 1991.

Clendening L. *Source Book of Medical History*. New York, NY: Paul B. Hoeber, Inc.; 1942.

Edgar II. *The Origins of the Healing Art. A Psycho-Evolutionary Approach to the History of Medicine*. New York, NY: Philosophical Library, Inc.; 1978.

Farrar GE Jr, Krosnick A. Wound healing. *Clin Ther*. 1991;13:430-434.

Forrest RD. Early history of wound treatment. *J R Soc Med*. 1982;75:198-205.

Forrest RD. Development of wound therapy from the dark ages to the present. *J R Soc Med*. 1982;75:268-273.

Haggard HW. *Mystery, Magic, and Medicine. The Rise of Medicine From Superstition to Science*. Garden City, NJ: Doubleday, Doran and Company, Inc.; 1933.

Lyons AS, Pertrucelli RJ II. *Medicine. An Illustrated History*. New York, NY: Harry N. Abrams, Inc.; 1987.

Majno G. *The Healing Hand. Man and Wound in the Ancient World*. Cambridge, MA: Harvard University Press; 1975.

Popp AJ. Crossroads at Salerno: Eldridge Campbell and the writings of Teodorico Borgognoni on wound healing. Historical vignette. *J Neurosurg*. 1995;83:174-179.

Rhodes P. *An Outline History of Medicine*. London, UK: Butterworths; 1985.

ACKNOWLEDGMENTS

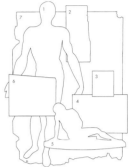

The publisher wishes to acknowledge the sources of the following photographs and illustrations:

Cover: 1 and 3, New York Academy of Medicine; 2, Hirmer Verlag, Munich; 4, University of Pennsylvania Art Collection, Philadelphia; 5, Museo Capitolino, Rome; 6, Städelsches Kunstinstitut, Frankfurt am Main; 7, Bibliotheque Nationale, Paris.

Text: Page 8, Clough/University of Pennsylvania Museum, Philadelphia; 9, Universitätsbibliothek, Leipzig; 10, World Health Organization, Geneva; 11, The Louvre, Paris; 13, The British Museum, London; 14, Museo Egizio, Turin; 15, Egyptian Museum, Cairo; 16-17, Wellcome Institute Library, London; 18-19, New York Academy of Medicine; 20, Archaeological Museum, Istanbul; 21, Bildarchiv Preussischer Kulturbesitz, Berlin; 22 & 30, Scala/Art Resource, New York; 23, Museo Capitolino, Rome; 24, Österreichische Nationalbibliothek, Vienna; 25, Bibliotheque Nationale, Paris; 27, The British Library, London; 28, Lilly Library, Indiana University, Bloomington; 31, Germanisches National Museum, Nürnberg; 32, Semmelweis Medical Historical Museum, Budapest; 33, National Library of Medicine, Bethesda; 34, Institut Pasteur, Paris; 36, Library of Congress, Washington; 37, Stanley B. Burns, MD and The Burns Archive; 38, Martin Bond/Science Photo Library; 39, Mongerson-Wunderlich Galleries, Chicago; 40, Johnson & Johnson, New Jersey; 41, D. McMullan/Science Photo Library; 45, SuperStock, Inc.; 46, James King-Holmes/Science Photo Library; 47, Tom Grill/COMSTOCK.